Diabetes 2

Top Foods to Help You Beat It

Naturally

Summary

This booklet provides general information on foods for people who are suffering from type 2 diabetes. When you have type 2 diabetes, it is necessary to make healthy food choices. Here, in this book we have listed out those healthy foods that you can use in order to reduce the complications and the austerity of this disease.

By selecting nutritious food items and being active, you can keep your blood sugar levels intact. Taking steps to manage your day-to-day diet, as mentioned in this guide, will help you a lot. Whether you are suffering from this condition or you want to know more about this or to care for somebody with this ailment, we hope that all the information available in this book will provide you with a great amount of help.

Table of Contents

What is Type 2 Diabetes?

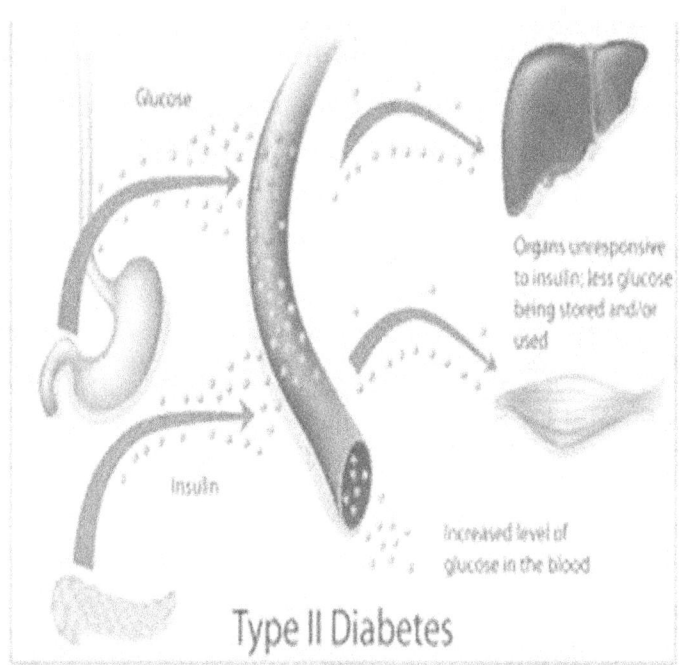

Type 2 Diabetes is a medical condition that can occur when the body is no longer able to manage the rising levels of sugar (glucose) in the blood. In this disease, the body stops producing sufficient insulin to deal with this resistance. Your body uses insulin to control the levels of glucose in blood.

If your body does not have enough insulin to take care of your needs, you may bear the pain of weak muscles, obesity, nausea, headache and other health problems.

Why You May Develop This Problem

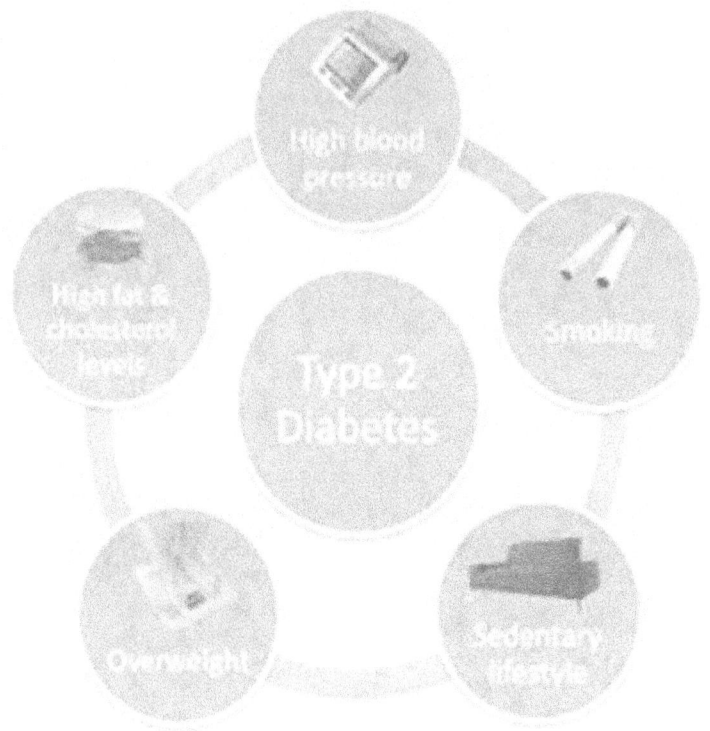

Type 2 diabetes can occur as a result of lifestyle and genetic factors. A sedentary lifestyle that uses fewer physical activities can particularly cause this problem to become worse.

Here we are going to list some of the key reasons why type 2 diabetes can occur in the human body:

Main Causes of Diabetes

Stress

Obesity

Overeating

Insulin resistance

High blood pressure

No physical activities

High level of cholesterol

Deficiency of insulin in body

Genetic and hereditary factors

Too much intake of sugar and oil

What Are the Warning Signs of Type 2 Diabetes?

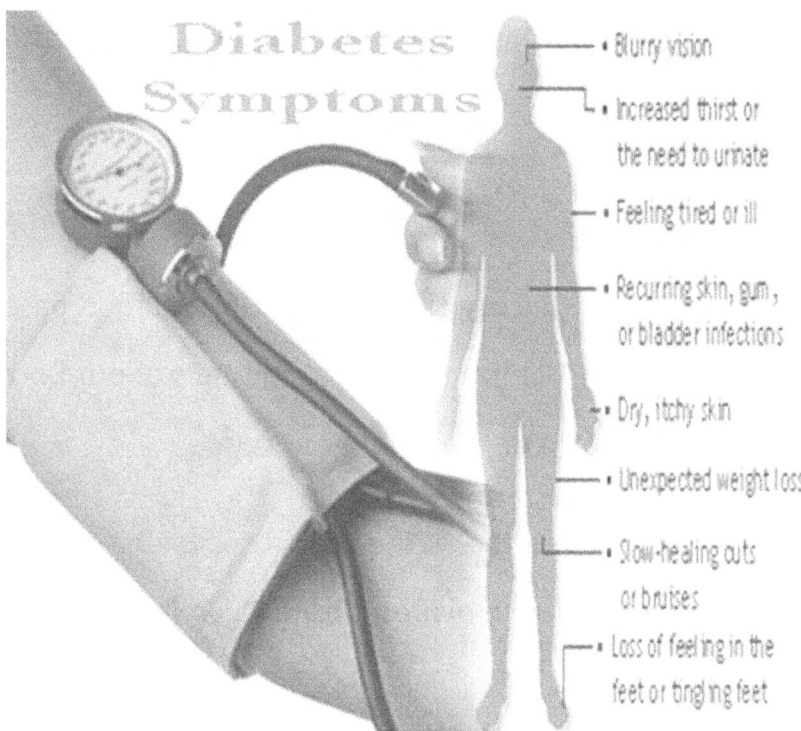

The signs of type 2 diabetes are closely linked with high levels of sugar in your blood.

Some of the common symptoms of type 2 diabetes are highlighted here:

Unquenchable thirst for liquids: If you are drinking excessive water, it could be a sign of type 2 diabetes.

Unexplained weight loss: This sign is more visible with type 2 diabetes. Without putting efforts, a diabetic person's body can cut down fat at a dangerously high rate due to an increase of insulin resistance in the body.

Fatigue and weakness: Glucose that we get through food passes into the bloodstream and insulin transfers it to the cells of our body. Blood cells use this insulin to provide us energy.

But, when the insulin is not there, the cells stops taking any action and due to this, a person with diabetes type 2 can feel exhausted and run down.

Other symptoms that can occur are-

Drowsiness

Blurred vision

Frequent urination

Slow healing of minor wounds

Frequent skin and bladder infections

Understanding the Complications

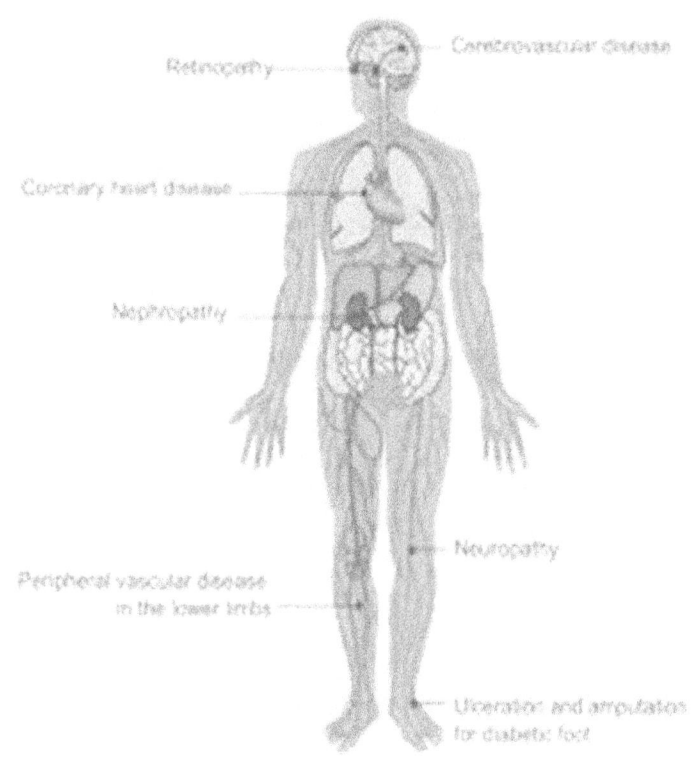

In order to get rid of type 2 diabetes, it is essential to take the right and timely treatment for this condition. If the disease is not treated on time; it can easily give birth to various health complications. High glucose levels in your body can damage your nerves, organs and blood vessels. Controlling your high blood sugar can help in the prevention of the complications that comes with this disease.

Risk of heart stroke and other diseases: Overflowing levels of glucose in your body augment the probability of atherosclerosis in your body. This condition results in a short supply of blood to the heart and often leads to heavy pains in the heart.

Nerve damage: Soaring levels of glucose in your body can easily damage small blood vessels. This can result in a burning sensation or tingling pain in your limbs. If the nerves are affected by glucose, you may bear complications like constipation, vomiting, headache and nausea. These nerves can also become damaged over time if they are not controlled properly.

Kidney disease: Your kidneys works in a less efficient manner if the tiny blood vessels in kidney get blocked due to glucose. In some cases, kidney diseases may even lead to kidney failure.

A Few Steps to Eating Well

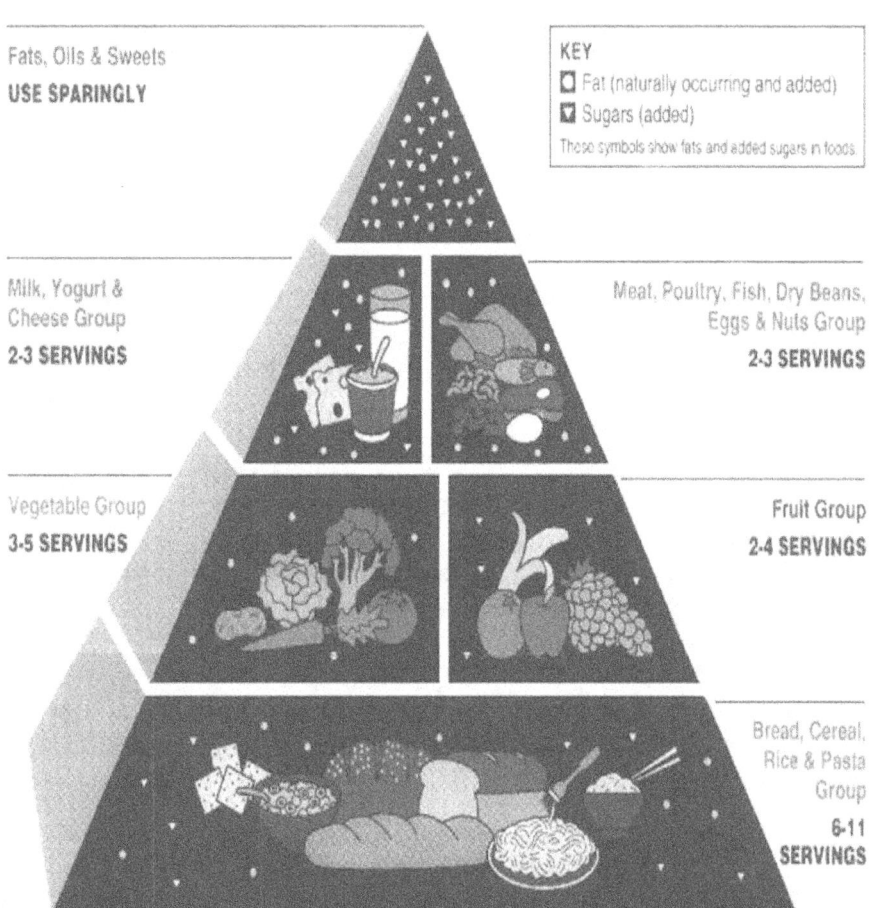

Take three meals in a day: Breakfast is the most important meal of the day so avoid skipping the first meal of the day. Divide your meals carefully so you can control your body's blood sugar levels to keep them in check.

Include starchy food with each meal: You must consume starchy carbohydrate-rich foods with all of your meals each day including your breakfast, lunch and dinner. The amount of carbohydrates in your diet will help you to control the level of glucose within your blood.

Reduce the amount of fat: You need to start with a low fat diet as it will help you to manage your diabetes and to help you control your weight. You must reduce the total amount of saturated fat in your diet as it is not only harmful but also because it can raise your bad cholesterol levels, which are also known as LDL. Go for lean meats instead of fatty meats. Choose low fat dairy products like semi-skimmed or skimmed yoghurt, milk and cheese spread.

Reduce the intake of salt: High levels of salt in your diet can increase your blood pressure and can cause you to be more likely to develop heart disease or a stroke. Reduce the amount of junk foods in your diet and stick with raw foods instead of processed stuff.

Eat more vegetables and fruits: Make it a rule to have at least five different fruits and vegetables in a day. By this your body will get sufficient minerals, vitamins and antioxidants and all these can help you in the fight against diabetes.

Before having breakfast, lunch or dinner, make sure you keep these simple guidelines in your mind to minimize the risk of type 2 diabetes in your body.

Top Foods to Reduce the Risk of Type 2 Diabetes

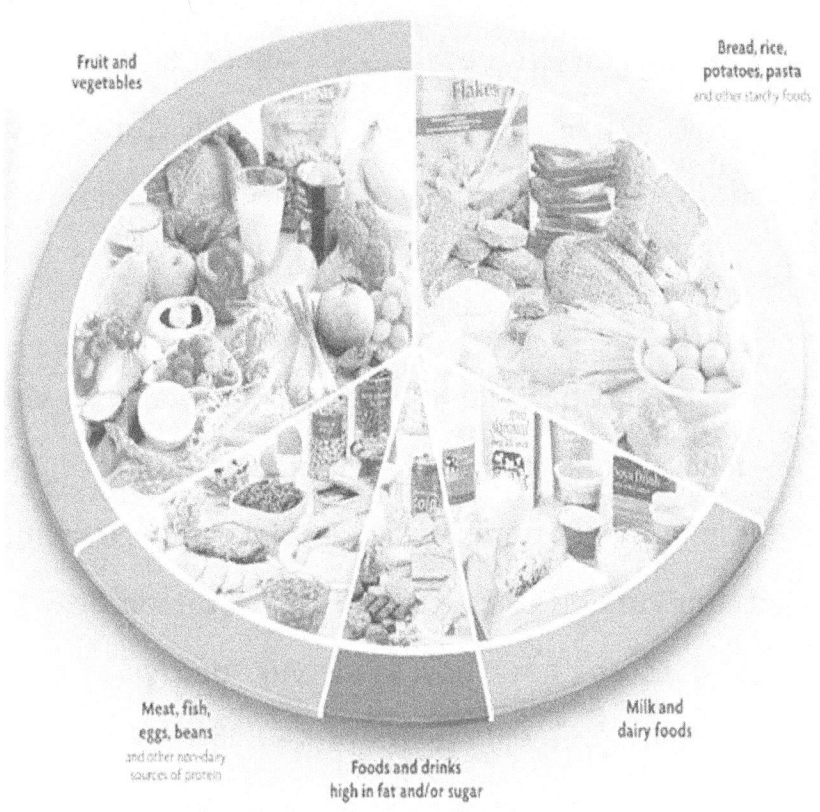

A well-balanced diet is essential for helping you to keep your risk for type 2 diabetes in check. Here, we are going to throw a light on the top foods that you should add in your diet. Including these power packed foods will reduce the risk of complications related to diabetes.

Blueberries: Savor the benefits of juicy blueberries by adding them in your pancakes and smoothies. These scrumptious berries are laden with vitamin C, flavonoids and dietary fiber. The flavonoid is a kind of phytonutrient that reduces the level of bad cholesterol and offers antioxidant protection to your body. About 3/4 of a cup of blueberries will contain around 15 grams of carbohydrates. In addition, this carb has the potential to your improve vision.

Beans: Beans are enriched with high fiber contents and a wonderful source of minerals and vitamins such as magnesium, potassium, folate and iron. All these antioxidants are necessary to maintain the right balance amid fluids like electrolytes. Try to add beans in your midday meal because these tiny seeds will load you with a good number of proteins. You will require protein in your body to repair worn out cells, building muscles and improve your bones to make them stronger and less likely to fracture.

Olive Oil: Also labeled as 'Liquid Gold,' olive oil slows down the likelihood of diabetes complications as it contains an anti-inflammatory component. The good fat in olive oil will not cause your body to resist insulin. A dash of this powerful oil can improve your digestion and thus the foods that you consume will not cause you to experience glucose spikes.

Broccoli: The nutritional power of this magical veggie can't be underrated. The non-starchy superfood has both vitamins A and C. These vitamins can work well to promote healthy bones, skin and teeth and can even improve your vision. These vitamins are also necessary for healing infections and wounds and can shield your body from a number of heart diseases.

Carrots: Raw or cooked, juicy carrots must be added in your diet to fight against diabetes. You can start your day with a fresh glass of carrot juice or you can add red carrots in your salad platter. Carrots are packed with beta-carotene, phytonutrients, carotenoids and vitamin A. Phytonutrients in carrots may help stop heart diseases and cancer.

Fish: Diabetes is one of the biggest causes for heart-related complications. Eating fish twice in a week can cut down your diabetes risk by approximately 40%. Herring, mackerel, sardines, tuna, salmon and trout are enriched with omega-3 fatty acids, which can help trim down the risk of diabetes complications like high blood pressure, clotting of blood, inflammation and the slow healing of wounds.

Cranberries- These yummy berries are power packed with vitamin C, anthocyanins and phytonutrients. Cranberries protect your body from the complications that takes place due to type 2 diabetes like urinary tract infections, slow healing of wounds and other cardiovascular diseases. You can take cranberry juice or add the juicy berries to salads and smoothies. If you buy pre-packed berries then be sure to check out the level of sugar in cranberry products as some products tend to come with unnecessary additives.

Apples: You must have heard an old adage that 'An apple a day keeps the doctor away". The axiom seems pretty relevant when you consider ways to keep type 2 diabetes under control or to avoid this problem. Delectable apples are filled with enough fiber and low in calories.

The high fiber content in this fruit can satisfy you for a long time. Eat apples without peeling them because the peel contains querctetin that has the potential to reduce the risk of type 2 diabetes due to its antioxidant effect.

Green Tea: Recent health studies proved that 2 cups of green tea in a day could do wonders for your overall health. Regular consumption of green tea reduces the likelihood of heart attacks and prevents the absorption of blood sugar in body. A simple and economical solution, green tea can fight issues that are related to diabetes. So sip this healthy beverage everyday and minimize the problems of diabetes.

Nuts: Filled with vitamin E, flavonoids, fiber, protein and monosaturated fats, nuts are best known to cut down the level of bad cholesterol. Nuts like hazelnut, walnut, almonds, pecans and macadamia are high in calories, but good for your heart. A regular intake of nuts lowers the risk of type 2 diabetes. You can munch dry nuts or sprinkle powdered nuts on your veggies, salads, yoghurt etc.

Oatmeal: A healthy breakfast alternative for morning, oatmeal has an adequate amount of fiber to keep you full for a long time. The natural goodness of soluble fiber in oats can reduce high blood pressure, normalize the levels of blood sugar in your body and improve digestion and lower bad cholesterol. Along with having good fiber content, oats also endow your body with potassium, magnesium and vitamins B and E, which may help lower the complications related to type 2 diabetes.

Spinach: Don't make a long face! Spinach is fibrous, filling and full of antioxidants. The dark green leafy veggie is packed with minerals and vitamins such as copper, magnesium, folate, fiber, zinc, potassium and vitamins like B2 and B6. The green vegetable has the potential to lessen the risk of diseases like diabetes, cancer, cataract and heart diseases. High in beta-carotene, spinach also shield the cells of body from harmful free radicals. Make sure you eat a small bowl of spinach everyday to keep diabetes symptoms away from you.

These are some nutritious foods that you need to add in your diet to fight efficiently against the symptoms of type 2 diabetes.

Meal Suggestions

If you have diabetes then you need to keep an eye on your plate. In order to make your eating habits balanced, it is necessary for you to make small changes in your diet plan. Use the below listed ideas to keep your sugar levels under control.

Breakfast Ideas

One glass of skimmed milk with a small banana or one boiled egg and brown bread with low fat spread and a glass of fresh orange juice is great to find. You can also start your day with bran flakes with low fat milk.

One cup low fat yoghurt and porridge with 1 dessertspoon of sultans can work but make sure that the yoghurt should be sugar-free.

Low fat milk or natural yoghurt with shredded wheat and strawberries can also give you plenty of filling stuff for your dietary needs.

Low fat milk and weetbix, ryvitas and marmalade with less sugar are all great to have.

Wholegrain toast with low fat spread and grilled tomato or poached egg is a good breakfast option.

Cracottes/crackerbread and low fat spread, low fat milk, a kiwi and oaotibix could help you out big time.

Lunch Ideas

For lunch, you can start with a fresh apple, one wholegrain bread slice with low fat cheese and homemade vegetable soup.

Another option is to use sweet corn with 1 tbsp low fat mayonnaise, a pita bread sandwich made with tuna and a slice of fresh melon to end up the meal.

The next option is freshly cooked pasta with chicken and tomato sauce. The sauce should be homemade. You can also take one cup natural yoghurt as curd can improve your digestion.

One pear can be used with baked beans and baked granary bread.

A small plate of salad with a small bagel and an omelet of two eggs with 1 tbsp of low fat oil is another choice.

Next, you can cook grilled mushrooms and rashers, nectarine/peach (if in season) and potato waffles.

Dinner Ideas

Your dinner can consist of mashed potatoes or carrots, or applesauce with a lean grilled pork chop.

One big size baked potato with low fat gravy can also be added. In addition, you can find roasted lamb with light fried cauliflower or broccoli.

Baked haddock/cod with black pepper and lemon juice, chopped mixed peppers with frozen peas and couscous is a healthy option to find.

Wholegrain rice with fresh vegetables and stir-fried chicken is another dinner choice to use.

One boiled or baked potato with a small bowl of vegetable or chicken casserole is a great option to go with.

There's also the option of having pasta with chili con carne and salad.

Baked noodles with frozen peas is a basic yet filling option. Fish lovers can also take salmon marinated for ½ hour in orange juice, soy sauce and garlic paste with wholegrain bread or rice.

Wholegrain rice one small bowl or two brown breads with boiled vegetables is the last option to have.

Snacking Ideas

Here are a few basic options to have when finding a quality snack:

One fresh fruit

One small cup low fat natural yoghurt

Cucumber, oat crackers/ rice cakes or crisp bread with low fat cheese spread and homemade tomato sauce

Low fat milk with a small bowl of cereal of your choice.

4 plain biscuits with a small cup of low fat milk or a small bowl of sprouts

You should also drink at least 8-10 glasses of water each day in order to take advantage of all of these ideas.

Healthy Eating Guidelines

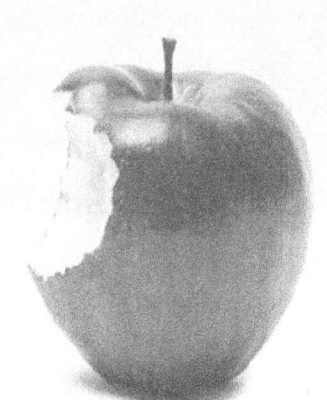

The main points about healthy eating are as follows:

Do not skip your meals. Take your breakfast, lunch and dinner on time and try to do it at the same time each day for the best results.

Include starchy carbohydrates such as potato, rice, cereal, pasta and bread in your daily diet.

Cut down your consumption of sugary and sweet foods.

Change the type of fat you take and reduce your fat intake.

Make it a rule to eat vegetables and fruits on a regular basis.

Eat fish once or twice a week. You can eat oily fish once in a week and baked fish with a little bit of salt twice in a week.

Cut down the intake of fast foods in your diet because processed food items can easily increase glucose levels in your body.

If you take alcoholic beverages, try not to take more than 5 standard beverages in a single sitting.

Regular Meals

As mentioned earlier, have your meals at regular times every day. If you feel hungry in the middle of your meals, you can have low fat yoghurt or a small bowl of fresh fruits of your choice.

Carbohydrates

Carbohydrates are a vital source of energy for your body and this food group has the potential to raise your blood sugar levels effectively. Carbs consist of starches and sugars. However, with diabetes it is necessary to select the right carbohydrates that help you to control your blood glucose levels.

The following foods are the prime source of carbohydrates:

Starchy Carbohydrates

Plantain/Yam

Noodles/Rice/Pasta

Cereals

Potatoes

Crackers and breads

Sugary Carbohydrates

All sweet foods, such as jams, non-diet fizzy drinks, chocolates, cakes, marmalades, biscuits and other sweet items.

Naturally Occurring Sugars

Fresh Fruits and fruit juices

Pulses and vegetables (lentils, beans and peas)

Dairy food (Yoghurt and milk)

While planning your diet plan to control your sugar levels, make sure you must add starchy foods in your each meal. Make sure you meals have the same amount of carbs in each as this plan can help to control glucose levels in your body. In order to increase the fiber content in your diet, try to use wholegrain varieties of these foods, e.g. brown rice, wholegrain bread, whole wheat pasta and wholegrain cereals. A sufficient amount of fiber in your daily diet ensures good digestion and healthy bowel functions.

Fats

Having type 2 diabetes augments your risk of heart related complications, but eating a reduced amount of fat can help you reduce your potential to develop such issues. Along with this, it is also essential for you to eat the right kind of fat.

How to Cut Down the Intake of Fat?

Instead of butter, choose a low fat spread.

Choose low fat dairy products, such as low fat yoghurt, low fat cheese and low fat milk.

Choose fat free dressings, low fat mayonnaise and low fat salad cream.

Instead of chocolates, tarts, crisps and cakes eat fruit, rice cakes, cereal with low fat milk, plain popcorn and low fat yoghurts.

Avoid deep frying and use healthy cooking methods, such as poaching, baking, steaming, boiling or microwaving.

Conclusion

Type 2 diabetes is a life-threatening disease, but with proper treatment and healthy eating habits, you can easily triumph over this medical condition. In this book, we have highlighted the important aspects related to diabetes like its prime causes, symptoms, ways to plan your meals to reduce its complications and many other important things. Here, we have penned down the foods that you should add in your daily diet to keep you from suffering from the effects of this condition.

We hope you liked all the suggestions mentioned in this simple guide!